Save His Heart

By: Krystal B. Parrish

For my strong & courageous son,

Kendryck!

You are my WORLD and I don't

know where I'd be if I weren't

your mommy!

Introduction

I wrote this book, "Save His Heart," to give hope to other parents going through battles of Congenital Heart Disease (CHD) with their child, or children. I only wish I had something like this when I found out my only son had this disease.

"Save His Heart" was also written to spread awareness for CHD. Many people aren't even aware that this excruciating disease even exists. Therefore, they are unaware of the dangers and trials it produces. I, personally, had never heard about it until my son was diagnosed shortly before he turned 3 months old.

"Save His Heart" is about a young single mother (myself) and her son's journey with this deadly disease. While giving the timeline of my son's battle, I also give extensive detail of my journey through these trying times.

I sincerely hope this book serves it's purpose and helps those on the same horrible road we were on. I believe if only one person is helped with this entirely true story, then I have done what God has called me to do... to inform other parents that there is hope out there.

I also want to let you all know that I only put one name, my son's name, in this book for a reason. "Save His Heart" was written to honor my son and I want it to stay totally and completely about him.

Furthermore, I dedicate this book to my son, Kendryck, for being so strong during his battle and making me a better person just by having him in my life. I also dedicate this book to my parents, other family and friends, and all of the medical professionals who helped my son and I through these extremely difficult and trying times.

Thanks for reading,

Krystal

<u>Chapter One</u>

At the time, I thought I had made an enormous mistake. I had just turned 19 years old and held a job as sales associate at the local superstore. I didn't even have the job long, just about two months. I wasn't ready to be a mom and I didn't think I would be a good one. The baby's father and I were no longer together and that left more fears and reservations dwelling inside me.

Today, however, I don't regret it at all. I honestly do not know where my life would have taken me if I hadn't become a mom. Motherhood has strengthened me in so many ways it is nearly unbelievable.

On March 25, 2008 at 11:45 a.m., God

blessed me with the most beautiful baby boy,

Kendryck. He was born weighing 7 pounds 2

ounces and measuring 19 1/2 inches long. Kendryck

was a perfect, healthy baby to have been born

nearly a month early, or so I thought.

His name was chosen from a baby name

book. First, it started with a "K" like mine. Second,

the name was different and unique. And third, I

thought it was cute.

I didn't really pay much attention to the

meaning of the name at the time. After all, I was

only 19 years old and, as you may well know,

teenage girls make their decisions on cuteness.

Kendryck means "bold." I like to believe

God gave me this name for him because it would

suit him greatly in his days to come.

My new son and I were discharged the day

after his birth because the doctors said we were both doing great. Kendryck was actually discharged before I was. We arrived home in the early evening and were greeted by loving relatives who were overjoyed Kendryck was finally here. Without looking through his baby book, though, I really couldn't tell you who all was there.

Everyone coming over showed me that my son and I were loved. This gave me a great reassurance that I could make it as a single mother. We had such a tremendous amount of love surrounding us so I knew if I ever needed anything, I could turn to any one of them.

During the first couple of months, everything seemed to be going fantastic! I loved being a mommy... even when I had to wake up every two hours for feedings. I was just so happy about having my son that nothing seemed to bother me. Before Kendryck, I had an extremely weak stomach when it came to changing dirty diapers. After he came along, though, I did it with pride!

It was weird. It was like the second he was born, I was programmed with all of this information on taking care of an infant. There were times, however, when I felt discouraged... like when he had colic and cried all night, or when I was just extremely tired. At these times, my parents would step in and help me.

I am so thankful to have had them and to have them in our lives. Anytime I needed someone they were there without question. The many trips to the hospital each time I went into labor, my mother by my side during delivery and my father standing outside the door, and lending a helping hand when I needed sleep or something. This was nothing compared to what they would do in the days ahead.

Through all the blissfulness of being a new mom with the most amazing baby boy, I was noticing some signs that weren't normal. Kendryck had difficulty breathing, his chest would cave in and his whole body would move with each breath, and he had projectile vomiting.

I took him to 2 pediatricians and a nurse practitioner before we finally settled with his current pediatrician. I knew the symptoms he was experiencing wasn't right, but I kept being told it was just because he was born too early and his lungs weren't developed yet.

Thoughts filled my mind. The main question was, "If his lungs weren't developed yet, why was he released from the hospital after his birth?" This didn't make any sense to me.

For his two month check up, I took him to a pediatrician I had wanted him to go to all along. I really expected to just be told the same thing once again. I thought we would just go in for the visit, the doctor would listen to his chest, he would get his shots, and we would be on our way. I guess I had been told that he was okay so much that it started settling in. Boy was I wrong.

I waited patiently at the end of the exam bed while his new pediatrician was listening to his breathing and I noticed he was listening longer than the other ones had before. He pulled the stethoscope from his ears and looked up at me with a quizzical look.

"Has anyone ever told you about him having a heart murmur?"

"No," I replied, scared out of my mind. I couldn't even manage to release any other words, though they were swarming my mind like bees. I wanted to ask him questions but I felt like someone had punched me in the chest and I couldn't breathe. I suddenly felt so sick!

The pediatrician explained to me that Kendryck had a very distinct heart murmur that is most likely caused by a hole in his heart. He said he was guessing it was a rather large hole because it (the murmur) was so loud. He explained the facts to me and I stood there, silent, trying to fight away the tears. I could tell he didn't want to tell me all the details but I asked him to. This piece of information was "need to know" for me. Could he die?

The answer was yes. I could lose my sweet

angel to this awful disease that I knew nothing about. In fact, death from this was common.

The pediatrician informed me that it normally took months to get into one of the best children's hospitals in the world, Texas Children's Hospital, but he would call every day until he got Kendryck in.

I left the doctor's office feeling numb. Holding Kendryck extra close, I walked to my car in a trance. I carefully buckled him in his carseat and kissed his tiny head and then I called my mom. She had went to the doctor with my younger sister that day. Through tears I managed to tell her what was going on, trying not to leave anything out, and she stayed on the phone with me until I calmed down.

On the drive home, I was in deep thought.

My family had a history of heart problems. My maternal great-grandfather died from heart disease. My grandmother (his daughter) had bypass surgeries. My mother (her daughter) was in the hospital for heart problems. There is also a history of heart problems on my dad's side. My paternal grandmother's brother had his first open heart surgery when he was 19 years old. My dad has an enlarged heart. My younger sister has Atrial Tachycardia.

I didn't have any heart problems, though. I had asthma when I was younger and when I was pregnant but that was it. Immediately, there were many thoughts of what I did wrong during my pregnancy. What did I do to make him sick like this?

Just so you know, I have always thought the

worst about every situation because when the worst doesn't happen, then I wouldn't be so disappointed or upset. So, I immediately thought the worst. I even used this technique during delivery. I thought I was going to die. That way, when I didn't die then the whole process wouldn't seem so hard and painful. Looking back, that technique is quite comical.

We made a stop on the way home to see a good friend. I thought she could make me feel better but the words she spoke didn't stick. They just went in one ear and out the other. But, she did try.

In the days to come, I did try to be patient and have faith. I searched heart murmurs and infants with holes in their hearts on the internet. I needed to know the facts.

Honestly, the facts didn't help out any. They

just made me feel worse. The facts just confirmed that my son could die like many other babies do because of this disease.

I called the doctor's office everyday to see if they had heard anything and everytime, they hadn't.

Finally, I got a call from the cardiologist's office. The receptionist set up a date and time for us to come in and have tests run to find out the source of his problems. The appointment was set for June 19th, 2008, just about a week and a half from that day.

Now it was just time to wait, again! But now we were waiting for that day to come. It seemed to approach slowly but when it finally arrived, I was more scared than when I went into labor the first time, 2 months early. It was time to find out just how bad his heart problems were... If he was going to overcome this problem and live a full life or

would his life be cut extremely short because of this

hole in his heart?

Chapter Two

June 19th arrived and I was finally going to find out what exactly was wrong with my baby. I would finally get the answers I needed.

My mother drove us to the appointment. Yes, I am very capable of driving myself but my mother knew that I needed the love and support of my mother there. And she also knew that if the cardiologist gave me bad news, I would be too distracted to drive in that much traffic. She knew I would be crying the entire way home.

The drive was two hours one way. I sat in the backseat with Kendryck because I didn't know how he would react to that long ride. Just for the record, he was not happy! He was content when the car was moving, but as soon as we stopped at a red traffic light or a stopsign, he became very fussy. We had to stop at a shopping center once so I could get him out and walk around with him. I guess it was good we left early.

Since we left so early, though, we arrived at the cardiologist's office an hour early and had to leave and go get lunch. I was a bit relieved that I didn't have to face the music, so to speak, right then. Mom, Kendryck, and I went to a pizza buffet restaurant and waited until time to go back.

When we went back, I noticed all the bright colors. It wasn't like a hospital. Hospital walls are mainly white and boring. I hate solid white walls! I'm not sure why actually. I sat in a doctor's office one time with solid white walls and no pictures or anything. That room made me so anxious to get out of there!

But this office had green, purple, blue, and

orange walls. I'm sure there were other colors, I just can't remember all the colors that were there. There was a television with cartoons playing, a "quiet room" with lots of books, and kids playing everywhere. Seeing this eased my anxiety a little because it was so informal. If Kendryck were old enough, he would have been down running around and playing, too.

We weren't sitting there long when a nurse called Kendryck's name. My heart jumped when I heard his name but I calmly got up and carried him to where she was. She lead us to a room with scales and a computer.

The nurse weighed Kendryck and then measured him. After that was finished, she checked his temperature, blood pressure, and his oxygen levels with the pulse oximeter.

When all of his vitals were taken, she lead us down a bright and colorful hall with pictures on the walls. The nurse showed us what room to wait in and then she left. Shortly after, a young man with curly hair walked in the door. He explained that he was Kendryck's cardiologist and they would be running a number of tests.

Truthfully, I can't remember what order the tests were in. I think the EKG (electrocardiogram) was first, and then chest x-rays, and last the echocardiogram.

The electrocardiogram, also known as EKG, is used for recording the changes of electrical potential occurring during the heartbeat. Of course, the x-rays are for taking pictures of his heart and lungs. I'm pretty sure everyone knows what x-rays are.

An echocardiogram is an ultrasound of the heart. It is a non-invasive technique involving the formation of a two-demensional image used for the examination and measurement of internal body structures and the detection of bodily abnormalities. I took these definitions out the dictionary so that I could better explain them to you.

With the EKG, the nurse took Kendryck's shirt off and hooked all these wires to his chest. A long slip of paper was printed out with a bunch of squiggly lines on it. This was the measurement of his heartbeat. It was hard for me to see all these wires hooked up to him whether it was temporary or not. Kendryck just layed there. I felt bad for him because he didn't understand what was going on and why he had all of those weird patches and wires on him. He looked at me with sad eyes and I could have burst into tears right there.

Kendryck didn't like the chest x-ray. He hates to be held down and two people had to hold him down to get a good enough picture for a sufficient reading. And for such a small child, it was pretty difficult for two of us to hold him still. I'm pretty sure everyone in that office heard him screaming.

Once it was over, I picked him up and he was fine. He calmed down immediately once he was cuddled next to me. Being in his mommy's arms solved everything for him. I wish it could have cured his illness, too.

Then came the echocardiogram. I was most familiar with this technique because I had just been pregnant and had to have ultrasounds, like any other pregnant woman. Kendryck didn't fight her either.

He just layed there while she moved the wand around on his tiny chest. We could see the screen with red and blue patches on it. This I was not familiar with. I had no clue what the red and blue were for. All I could do was sit through it and wait for the cardiologist to explain them to me.

After his echocardiogram was finished, we were lead back to the room we were in before to wait on the doctor. It was only a few minutes until he waltzed gracefully into the room.

The cardiologist told me the tests proved that Kendryck had 4 holes in his heart. Two in the wall between the atrial chambers and two in the wall between the ventricle chambers.

These were labeled as Atrial Septal Defects (ASD) and Ventricular Septal Defects (VSD). The cardiologist informed me that two of the holes were tiny enough that, on their own, they didn't matter. The third was a little larger and the other was about the size of a dime. He pulled his stool over in front of me to where his knees were touching mine and drew a diagram on a sheet of paper to better explain his diagnosis.

The cardiologist then explained to me what the red and blue patches on the echocardiogram indicated. Because of the larger holes, blood was backflowing through the holes and into his lungs. Kendryck's heart murmur had a very loud roar because there was a tremendous amount of blood pouring through the holes. To put it simply, his lungs were filling with blood.

Instead of just doing surgery, the cardiologist wanted to try medicines first. I was pleased with this. He explained that it would be better to wait because Kendryck was so little. The bigger the baby, the less the risk. He said he hoped the medicines would cause tissue to grow around the holes so they would grow up themselves. However, if the medicines didn't work, he would need surgery. I wasn't pleased with this.

We left the room and went down the hall to schedule his next appointment. I got the paper for his next appointment and exited the office. Once again, I felt numb. My mom called my dad and other family members to let them know what was going on. I can't remember calling anyone. Maybe I did. I know I sent text messages to friends who asked me to let them know but I can't remember actually talking on the phone. I can't remember even speaking a word.

We stopped to get the baby's medication and

I fed him while we were waiting. That was a time
we both loved. I loved holding him close to me and
stopping his tears (because, of course, he cried
when he was hungry) and he really loved to eat!
This was definitely a time I needed to hold him
close. My heart hurt just thinking about what he was
going to have to go through. Before long, the
feeding was over and we were on our way back
home.

Once back home, I searched Congenital
Heart Disease facts. I received information from the
cardiologist's office about a group called, "It's My
Heart," so I went to their website to find all of the
information I needed.

Congenital Heart Disease means he was
born with the heart disease. I learned that twice as
many kids die from CHD than all forms of

childhood cancers. There are so many different types of CHD out there and more are being discovered all the time. Now, my sweet angel was one of those statistics. He had one of the most common types though.

I actually tried staying positive this time but it didn't work. I found myself doubting God. This is expected with any mother, though. I mean, you're all excited about having a new baby and then, all of a sudden, you're finding out your baby has an awful disease he could die from.

The internet and, "It's My Heart," helped me learn everything I needed to know about Congenital Heart Disease. I read blogs, I read articles, I watched videos. Most of the videos, though, scared me beyond imagination.

The videos were like blogs of different

babies and their journeys through CHD. Most of them lost their battle. A few were still going but still having surgeries. I sat up countless nights crying profusely while watching these.

The possibility of death and the surgery was the hardest for me to handle. I have never been one to take death lightly. It has always been hard on me to lose someone I love. We lost my big brother when I was 10 years old and I knew how bad that hurt for me and my other siblings. But I also saw how horrible it was for my parents to lose a child. I wasn't certain how I would be able to handle that trial. I wasn't certain I could handle it all.

Crying was something I did more often than anything. A lot of nights, I found myself lying in bed just watching him sleep in his bassinet next to me. His little body fighting for each breath.

Every little thing scared me. The first time I woke up and realized he hadn't woken me up at all during the night and it was after 7 in the morning, when he normally woke up, I jumped out of bed and looked at him. I could see his body moving with each breath and was relieved that he was still with me.

Every time he cried, I ran to him. Every time he coughed, I ran to him. Every time he made a noise, I ran to him. People kept telling me I needed to stop that because he would be spoiled but I didn't care. How can you really care about spoiling your baby when you may not have them later? If he were to join the other angel babies in the sky, I wanted him to know his mommy loved him unconditionally and would do anything for him.

After a while, I built up a strong faith that

the medication would work. I just knew our next visit with the cardiologist was going to be a good one. He would run all the tests again and find that the medicines, or in my beliefs, God, had healed him.

I continued to give him the two medications each day like clock work and convinced myself that the next appointment would confirm my thoughts.

I was so sure that the cardiologist would tell me Kendryck was healed that I wasn't even really worried about this visit at all. He wouldn't need more medicines, he didn't need surgery, and he most definitely would not die. Once again, I was proved wrong.

Chapter Three

For the next visit, I felt even more confident while on the two hour drive. I was actually feeling excited because I knew in my heart he was okay.

We arrived and I signed him in and waited, like before, only this time with a huge smile. Shortly after, a familiar voice called Kendryck's name. It was the same nurse from the last visit. She greeted us with smiles and played with Kendryck. Then, she weighed and measured him and took his vitals, just like the last visit.

When she had completed her tasks, we were lead to an exam room to wait for the cardiologist. He came in and spoke with us and I remember thinking what a great doctor he was. A lot of doctors these days are "in and out" and don't really seem to care... at least in my experiences. But he always asked how we were doing and shared stories of his family with us. He always made us laugh.

After visiting for a few minutes, the cardiologist told us they were going to run the tests again and see if there were any improvements. So we went through everything again and when we got to the echocardiogram, we were greeted by another friendly face. We sat and talked for a few minutes until she had everything ready to go and even some during the procedure.

I noticed, though, the red and blue patches were still on the screen. Immediately, I felt drained and terrified. And again, I felt sick. When I turned to my mom, she verified with a look that she saw it, too. From that moment, I knew I was wrong. He hadn't been healed.

The cardiologist confirmed my recent suspicions. Kendryck was not healed. The medicines weren't working so he decided to increase his dosage.

His cardiology visits became more frequent and with each visit, the doctor explained that Kendryck's condition was worsening.

At one visit, the cardiologist noticed that the lasiks was taking too much salts out of Kendryck's body so he had to put him on yet another medication.

At one point, with prescriptions and over-the-counter medications, Kendryck was on 12 different medicines each day.

Our days were planned around medicine times. I had to set an alarm clock for each medicine time so I wouldn't get behind. Some of those medicines were at two or four in the morning. Life was pretty exhausting but it was keeping my baby with me.

We also had to take extra precautions such as making sure he was cool enough, he had enough fluids, he ate enough. I had to start putting extra formula in his bottles because he wasn't gaining weight like he was supposed to. The cardiologist said we needed to try everything to get meat on his bones so he even told me to start having cereal in his bottles early on, as well as giving him baby food.

At one of the last visits, the cardiologists told me the medicines were working. There was flesh growing. The only problem was it was growing in the wrong place. It had grown to where it was partially blocking one of his valves.

So, now he had 4 holes in his heart and a partially blocked valve.

By this time, I had lost all hope. I was absolutely distraught. I quit going to church and frankly was quite angry with God.

As I said before, I do not handle death, or even bad situations, very well. I was in a serious trance for a long time. All I did was go to work for a couple of hours a day, five days a week and then come home and spend all my time with my son. Missing a moment with him was not going to happen.

Actually, if infants could talk, he would have probably told me to leave him alone, quit kissing him so much, and quit taking so many pictures! I took pictures and kissed him constantly because I wanted as many as possible of each incase there came a time when I couldn't get them anymore.

In August, just two months after his diagnosis, I took Kendryck to his pediatrician for a routine check-up and shots. That was on a Friday afternoon. Over the following weekend, Kendryck got really sick and was running an extremely high temperature. First, I thought it was because of the shots but it just continued through each day. Of course, I alternated tylenol and motrin to keep the fever down but it would just come back and climb even higher. Monday morning, he was still running a fever so I called his pediatrician so I could get him an appointment.

The nurse managed to get him in right away so we left immediately. I thought maybe he was teething, or even had a summer cold. But when his pediatrician listened to his breathing, he told me to load him up and take him straight to Texas Children's emergency room. He said he would call and let them know I was on my way. He then explained to me that Kendryck had a lot more fluid in his lungs than he had had just the Friday before. So, complying with doctor's orders, I loaded him up and my mom and I sat out for the hospital.

Chapter Four

Upon arrival, the nurses were waiting so we didn't have to sit in the waiting room. I was happy with the way they were treating Kendryck and taking care of him so quickly.

In the triage room, the nurse took his vitals and hooked him to the pulse oximeter, which measures the amount of oxygen he's getting. The numbers weren't even going up to the 80s so they switched the machines out, thinking that would be the problem. When they hooked him to the other, however, they were getting the same reading. So, obviously, he wasn't getting enough oxygen.

The nurses moved him into a regular room, still in the emergency unit, and hooked Kendryck up to oxygen immediately. Then it was time to hook him to an IV.

This is the part where I got angry. The nurses wouldn't let me feed Kendryck because they were afraid he would aspirate so he was becoming dehydrated, which means it's hard to get a vein.

Maybe I was stressed, but I don't think any mother would have been happy with this situation. When it was all said and done, Kendryck had been poked 16 to 18 times before they finally got an IV in. I was livid! I ended up stepping out of the room and letting my mom take over because I couldn't stand seeing him like that. He had such pain in his eyes and it was like he was pleading with me to make them stop.

I did end up getting an attitude with them and telling them if they couldn't do it, then they needed to stop trying. My mom told them they needed to let me feed him, but they didn't let me.

After I was done griping at them, they went to get an older man who they said was experienced with finding the veins regular nurses couldn't. Sure enough, he was experienced. The male nurse had a successful IV stick in one try.

After all the chaos in the emergency room, Kendryck finally fell asleep from crying so hard. I had never felt more horrible in my life! I sat on the side of his bed and held his hand and without realizing, I fell asleep, too.

My mom, who is pretty much always with me, woke me up when the doctor came in. He was a young doctor who couldn't be older than 25. I think he was a first year resident or something.

This doctor informed me he had been in contact with Kendryck's regular cardiologist and that he had asked for him to explain everything to me. I was absolutely mortified by what he told me.

You know those movies where they slow the film down and the words that are spoken are really long and drawn out? That's how everything sounded to me. I swear I could hear my heart beating just as loud as the words he was speaking. It also felt as if all the breath had been taken from me.

Kendryck was going into congestive heart failure. There was a lot of fluid around his heart and the blood that was still backflowing was filling his lungs.

The young doctor informed me that lungs are like sponges... When they continue to be filled with liquid they quit working as well until eventually they quit working at all.

Kendryck was admitted to the hospital and

moved to the 15th floor. The doctor informed me that he would only be in overnight for observation and then he would have to go back for a check up with his cardiologist.

By the time we were moved upstairs, it was getting dark. Kendryck was still sleeping good so it made the move easier. My mom left to go back home and get some things we needed and told me she would be back the next morning. So there I was, in a silent hospital room with my sweet baby sleeping like the angel he was.

A young male nurse brought me formula, diapers, and wipes for him and made sure I was okay. I felt a little more at ease once we were settled in his room and once I could feed him as often as usual.

All through the night, the nurses came in

and checked his vitals but he continued to sleep good. He woke up once to eat and to have me hold him for a while and then he went back to sleep.

The next morning, a new nurse came in to try to take him off of the oxygen. She would turn it down little by little and he was fine, but when she cut it completely off, he could not get enough oxygen. It was the early evening before she could get him completely off of the oxygen but it was determined that he was going to need an inhaler.

A spacer and an inhaler were brought to me and the nurse showed me how to use it. Just for the record, Kendryck didn't like it at all! He would hold his breath when the spacer was placed over his face.

Finally, he was discharged and we were headed home for a couple of days before returning to his cardiologist for a check up.

Both of my parents accompanied me on this visit because we kind of suspected talk of surgery. Again, tests were ran and we were back in the room waiting on the cardiologist. Waiting was something I had to do constantly during this process but I was still impatient.

My parents were sitting in the two chairs by the door and I was standing up by the exam bed playing with Kendryck when the cardiologist entered. My mom took Kendryck so I could give the doctor my attention when he started giving me the results.

The cardiologist turned to me and started relaying information as if he were reading out of a book or re-enacting a movie scene. Kendryck's condition wasn't getting any better. In fact, it was getting worse.

I asked if the surgery could be done through his leg because I had read that some were done that way. The answer was no. There was no other option but open heart surgery.

I looked at Kendryck. He was sitting in his grandma's lap so innocent and had no clue what was going on. Even though I tried to fight them, I could feel the tears welling in my eyes and then they were just rolling down my face. The tears were uncontrollable, unstoppable.

The cardiologist, who was standing next to me, reached over, put his arm around me, and gave me a hug. He said he was going to run Kendryck's case before the board and see if they wanted to go ahead and do the surgery or let him stay on medication for a little longer. But even though, he was going to run it by them, he said it was best to do the surgery. Kendryck's condition just kept worsening and his lungs were deteriorating. If something wasn't done soon, his lungs would completely shut down.

We chatted for a while and the cardiologist told us to take all the time we needed to take everything in. I held Kendryck in my arms and my dad hugged me while I cried. I couldn't stand being in the room much longer. I had to get out of there.

The cardiologist informed us he would give me a call in about two weeks to let me know what was going to happen, so the wait was on again.

Chapter Five

During these times, it seemed when something happend, something else that was bad was right around the corner. Since we live in Southeast Texas, hurricanes are inevitable. On September 12th, we were hit by a category 2 hurricane. My mom was a dispatcher at the sheriff's office and had to work so my dad, Kendryck, and I stayed home during the storm. It seemed to last forever. In actuality, it lasted about 8 hours.

I remember sitting with Kendryck laying next to me and constantly checking if he was cool enough. We had lost power around midnight and since it was September, it was pretty hot. I sat shielding him from any harm, listening to the tornadoes all around the house, the sound of trees falling, and debris hitting this windows.

The storm progressed as the night did and it was getting more intense. We could hear the windows buckling and dad and I decided we needed to find a safer place to hunker down. I blocked the window in Kendryck's room and layed him in his crib while we went all over the house searching for the right spot.

Our home wasn't big, one story 4 bedroom 2 bathroom, but we had to weigh all factors. Windows, doors, etc.

Between going through each room, I went back to check on Kendryck just to make sure he was still okay and still cool. First, we tried Dad's music studio (which was converted from one of the bedrooms). There was a small bathroom in that room but there was also a window and it was on the end of the house. Next was the kitchen. There was a

window on one end and the back door on the other.
Then the living room which was already out
because of the front door and 3 large windows (and
it was where we started). His and Mom's room had
three windows also. My room had two windows.
Kendryck's room had a large window.

We finally ended up closing all the doors to
the bedrooms and putting the sofa cushions in the
hallway to sleep. I couldn't sleep though. Not just
because of the storm. I was worried about
Kendryck.

Shortly after we lost power, we lost cell
phone signal, too. Tornadoes had knocked down all
of the towers. So, if something happened to him I
couldn't call for emergency assistance.

I finally fell asleep for about an hour and
when I awoke, Kendryck was still sleeping and I

was looking up at the sky! My dad wasn't lying down anymore so I went to find him. He was in the house surveying the damage. A tornado had split our roof, which is why I saw the sky when I woke up. The kitchen had water all over the floor and the ceiling had fell through in half of his studio.

I walked back in the living room and pulled back the curtain to see the damage outside. When I looked out I couldn't help but think, "This resembles what has happened to our lives." Everything was torn apart. Damaged. Broken. It was awful.

Kendryck and I stayed with a very nice couple that night. The man was a police officer and he and his wife were friends of my parents. They knew about Kendryck's heart condition and offered their guest bedroom for us for the night. I was, and

still am, truly grateful to have them in our lives.
They had a large generator to power their home and
I was able to keep Kendryck comfortable. Kendryck
cut his first tooth that night at their house.

The next day my parents picked us up and
although I was sad to go I knew they would be a
part of our lives forever. I will forever feel a sense
of debt to them for opening their home, and their
hearts, to us to make sure my son was safe.

We ended up staying with my grandmother
in her one bedroom home after that night. Kendryck
needed a fan on him and she had a generator that
her brother, my great-uncle, had brought over. I
kept the same routine of medicines with Kendryck
and, again, had to wait for power to come back up.

In a way, I was glad we didn't have power or
cell phone signal because the cardiologist couldn't

call me to tell me Kendryck had to have surgery.

But I also knew without the surgery he wouldn't

make it.

A little less than a week after the storm, we

regained cell phone signal and I was able to call the

cardiologist's office. They only had my home phone

number so I had to be the one to make the initial

call.

Making the initial call was a difficult task

for me. Again, I was terrified and felt sick. I knew

when I called they would be talking to me about

cutting my son's chest open so to it's safe to say, I

was apprehensive.

I spoke with the nurse and she informed me

that she would call back when she spoke with the

cardiologist.

Some family friends were over visiting

when she called back. We were all sitting on the back porch at my grandma's when my cell phone rang. My heart jumped when I saw it was the cardiologist's office and everyone looked at me as if silently asking if it was the nurse. I answered, already having that golf ball in my throat feeling that you get when you're about to cry.

Of course, she told me yes, Kendryck had to have open heart surgery and she gave me the number to call and set up a date and time for a consultation with the surgeon. I put the number in my friend's (who is more like an aunt) phone and then hung up. I told everyone what the nurse said and then dialed the number she had given me. The apprehensive filled me again because once more, I had to be the one to make the initial call.

I spoke to a really nice lady who seemed

very understanding of my feelings. She set up the consultation for October 2nd, 2008, which was less than a month away. I hung up the phone, and again, told everyone what she said.

I didn't cry then, though. Kendryck was napping inside (the backdoor was open so I could see him). I calmy walked inside and layed down on the mattress next to him. He was in just a diaper to keep him cooler and I ran my finger down his chest, knowing his tiny chest would be cut open in just a few weeks. That's when I cried.

I thought I would never stop crying. I can't even begin to tell you how scared I was and how awful I felt that he would have to endure all this pain. I was 20 years old and had never had a surgery in my life and now my angel, 6 months old, was about to have his first surgery... and a major one at that.

I found myself running my finger down his chest just about every night. I would just lay there and stare at him and sometimes cry. Sometimes I whispered in his ear, telling him I loved him and I would be by his side through everything. I also told him I was sorry he had to go through this and if I could, I would take his place in an instant. And I told him I needed him to be strong and to fight... not to give up because I wasn't giving up on him.

I never told anyone but I was still angry with God through all of this. I did go to a few churches with my mom, though, and had them pray for Kendryck. Even though I was angry, I knew prayer worked. My prayers may not have worked when I asked God to heal him without surgery but I knew prayer had worked for people before and it was still working for people. And I knew some people with very strong faith and who could probably make mountains move, if they wanted. They were very Godly people and I knew if anyone's prayer would work, it would be their's.

October 2nd arrived. Kendryck and I were still staying at my grandma's and my parents were staying at our house. It was too unsafe for Kendryck.

I woke up that morning, got our mattresses picked up, fed Kendryck and myself and dressed him in this extremely cute outfit. Blue Jeans, a t-shirt, a pullover vest, and tennis shoes. He was so adorable.

I sat there for a while playing with him, having our "Mommy and Me" time, and taking pictures of him. We met my parents over at our house and set off for the surgeon's office, which was an hour away.

I was really glad I remembered the stroller because the surgeon's office was on the 20th floor. When we got off of the elevator, there were heart decorations everywhere and more "It's My Heart" posters and pamphlets.

We entered the lobby through huge glass doors and then were pointed in the direction of the right desk, down a long hall.

I signed Kendryck in and the receptionist pointed to a room for us to wait in. We waited for a short while when a nurse came in and told us to come with her. I didn't know he would be seeing a nurse here but he was. They measured him, weighed him, and took his vitals. Then he had to have another EKG.

When everything was taken care of, the nurse lead us to a different room. There were couches and chairs and pictures of babies who had had open heart surgery. Just looking at the photos mortified me!

My mind wandered. In just a few short weeks, I would be standing next to a hospital bed like that and my son would be the baby with his chest cut open. I immediately felt sick, a feeling that I had often since June 5th, the day I found out he had a heart murmur.

Not being able to look at the photos any longer, I returned to my chair and made Kendryck a bottle. I just wanted to cuddle him because I was scared. I wanted to just take all the problems and go through the surgery for him. But we all know that isn't possible.

My parents, Kendryck, and I waited quite a while before the surgeon came in. He introduced himself and shook our hands. Then he looked at Kendryck's chest. He wanted to see how it caved in.

The surgeon was a gentle, nice man. He spoke softly and was sure to answer all of the questions we had, which were numerous. A few of the questions were:

*What is the survival rate?

*Would this be the only surgery he needed?

*How long would he be in the hospital?

*Would he have any life long problems after the surgery?

The surgeon informed me that Kendryck's form of Congenital Heart Disease was actually very common and they expected there to be no problems with his surgery. He also said there was about at

99% chance Kendryck would never have to have another surgery, he would be in the hospital about a week if there were no complications, and he shouldn't have any problems from the surgery.

I handed Kendryck over to my mother as it came time to sign papers. My hands trembled. I had to give consent for a stranger to cut open my baby's chest. Again, I cried.

Before long, we were headed back home with heavy hearts. I took several pictures of him with my cell phone (one of which is the photo on the cover of this book). I attached the photo from the book cover to a text message that said, "Operation: Pray for Kendryck," and had a brief description of what was going on. The text spread among my friends and their friends. Later, I made a flier and it was passed around on the internet.

I can't express enough how scared I was that I was going to lose him. Kendryck, on the other hand, continued to be a normal, loving baby despite his illness. He loved to cuddle and just be held. I knew he had no idea what was going on so I was scared for him, too.

In the next two weeks to come, I tried to prepare myself for what was coming but it was impossible. I would lay next to him nearly every night running my finger up and down his chest because I knew there would be a scar there forever, if he survived.

Though I was angry with God, still, I took Kendryck to several different churches for prayer. Deep inside, I believed that God could and would heal him before he had to have the surgery. There were lots of prayers. There were lots of tears. But each morning I woke up, his tiny chest still caved in and nothing had changed.

The night before surgery arrived quickly. I had nothing packed and it was time for bed. My grandmother watched Kendryck for me so I could go next door to my parents' house and get our things ready. I didn't know exactly what to pack. I needed clothes for Kendryck, clothes for me, diapers, wipes, bottles, medicine, security objects, pacifiers, baby food, etc. To say I was stressed is an understatement.

At the consultation I was told I could put whatever I wanted in the bed with him after his surgery. I chose an object my Nannie (maternal great-grandmother) had bought me for Valentine's Day when I was a teenager. Nannie played an enormous role in our lives. She helped my parents raise us when we were small children because they worked so hard to provide a great life for us. Nannie loved Kendryck dearly, too. He was the 5th generation and she loved to spoil him. Nannie couldn't be at the hospital that day due to her breaking her hip so I wanted something from her there.

The object was small. It was in a clear and red container and contained a tiny vase inside that said "I love you" and had little roses in it. I also chose a picture from my first mother's day. Kendryck was about a little over a month old and I was holding him in front of a small fish pond at my maternal grandmother's home.

The day the picture was taken, on Mother's Day, was also the day Kendryck was dedicated to the Lord. So it was a double special day for us. It was before talk of heart murmurs, holes, blocked valves, and surgery. It was a time when we were just blissfully happy.

I had put the object from Nannie in the bag and before putting the picture in, I froze in place, just staring at the picture... Wishing I could go back to this day before my world came crashing down.

I'm guessing my mother saw that it was coming because she went to get my dad. They both returned to the living room and watched me for a minute and then before I knew it, there it was. The reality had hit and I had my first real breakdown.

My dad immediately grabbed me in his arms and my mom soon followed. I cried and I screamed until it was all out and I couldn't cry anymore. Maybe it was what I needed. Maybe I needed to just be held by my parents, who mean everything to me and who had done everything they possibly could for me, and just cry.

When my breakdown was over, I headed back over to my grandmother's to finish packing and get some rest. I was exhausted but every time I would lay down, I would remember something that I didn't pack. It was around 3 or 4 a.m. when I finally fell asleep and I had to wake up at 5 a.m.

Obviously, when it was time to get up, I was exhausted. It was a long trip to the hospital, though, and I knew I could get squeeze in a little more sleep. After all, I knew I wouldn't be getting much once we arrived at the hospital, our new home for a little while.

I dressed Kendryck in this black, long-sleeved onesie and a pair of jeans. The onesie was designed like the front of a tuxedo and said, "All dressed up." He was absolutely gorgeous.

We had to be at the hospital at 7 a.m. to get checked in and get Kendryck ready for surgery.

Mom, Dad, Kendryck, and I returned to the 20th floor and started the process. Again, I am so very thankful to have my parents. I was perfectly capable of doing things on my own but they knew I needed them. More than that, they wanted to be there. A parent's love is unexplainable. It is unconditional. A grandparent's love is about ten times that!

The process seemed to take forever. Kendryck was changed into a baby's hospital gown and he only wanted his grandpa. The tests were a little different from before. I think another EKG was performed but there were also blood and urine cultures.

Kendryck did not like the urine culture at all. They had to do something like a catheter because he wouldn't potty in the little bag. I, for one, didn't like this. I remembered how painful the catheter was from when I was pregnant but they stuck the tube in my baby boy and I did not like that! It made me hurt with him.

Once back on the 20th floor, we were directed to follow a young lady. She showed us everything we needed to know about the hospital. Where the surgery would take place, the CVICU (Cardiovascular Intensive Care Unit), where we would wait during surgery, and where he would be before surgery. She showed us the food court down stairs and the floor he would be on after he was released from CVICU and she showed us the Ronald McDonald housing and got us registered for a room.

After returning back to the 20th floor, we were able to get a break for lunch so it was back down to the food court. The time we had for lunch seemed to fly by so quickly. After lunch, the wait was once more.

Thankfully, the room we were waiting in was comfortable. It wasn't a normal waiting area. It was a private room with warm colors and low lights, 2 small couches and two or three chairs. We waited for a pretty long time up there. Long enough that we all fell asleep. It was no doubt we were exhausted from the morning's itenirary and just knowing there was so much more to come didn't help.

Kendryck was sleeping soundly on my chest, as he did many many times and I fell asleep just holding onto him.

Mom and Dad fell asleep on the couches adjacent from each other. I'm not really sure how long we were sleeping when a lady came in. She was the social worker for our case. When I heard she was a social worker, I thought I was in trouble for Kendryck being sick. Come one, I was 20 years old and had never heard of any other kind of social workers, except for the ones that come and take your kids away when you aren't a good parent.

But this social worker was here to make sure we had everything we needed and we had a counselor, if needed, and all that. She was also there to make sure we fully understood the process of what was going to happen and how long we would be there, etc. The social worker promised she would

be visiting us once we were settled on the 15th

floor, the "heart unit."

Finally, it was time to be moved to a regular room where we could have some quiet time and prepare for the following morning. I was given baby food, formula, diapers, and wipes once more even though I had brought enough for a month and I put everything up where it needed to be.

The room had a giant steel crib in the middle of the floor and all the usual gadgets you'd see in a hospital room. There was a couch that pulled out to a bed, a chair, a built-in desk and a tv with a playstation attached. The nurse's station checked out games to families staying there for free. I was never big on video games but it was something to do to occupy my time when Kendryck was sleeping.

He didn't sleep this time when we entered the room, though. He was sporting a diaper and his black t-shirt stating, "I'm with the band," and

playing with his mommy and grandparents. He was

a happy boy until the nurses came in to start an IV.

It was time to start preparing for surgery.

Before they even started the IV, I

interrogated them like I was a police officer and

they were suspects. I wanted to know their success

ratings on starting IV's and if they couldn't get a

vein, how many times they would try.

I liked these nurses because they informed

me that they were normally pretty good at getting

IV's but if they couldn't get one after three sticks,

they would stop and wait an hour or two before they

tried again.

I was pleased with this because I knew

Kendryck needed the IV but he didn't have to

endure so much pain. Thankfully, though, they were

able to get a good stick on the first or second try.

Kendryck cried for a little bit but as soon as the nurses were finished wrapping it up, I gave him a baby rice cake and it seemed to take away all the pain; or at least took his mind off of it. He was back to being a happy baby.

My parents stayed until later that evening and then went to stay with my dad's first cousin who lived near the hospital. I was a little edgy with them leaving because I had been used to their company but I knew they needed rest as much as I did.

The night seemed to last forever, which would have been fine with me, but Kendryck was not happy anymore. I wasn't allowed to feed him after midnight and only clear liquids until 5 a.m. The nurses supplied me with the clear liquids I needed for him and a couple more bottles to use.

I felt really bad for Kendryck because he was so hungry and wanted to eat but his surgery was scheduled for 7 a.m. so it was necessary for him to fast. I scheduled his last formula feeding to where it would end at midnight and his last clear liquids bottle to end at 5 a.m. to hold him over as best as possible.

My parents and my paternal grandmother arrived just before the sun came up. Now, we had to wait yet again, for them to come bring Kendryck back for surgery.

7 a.m. came and no one came for him. As 8 a.m. approached, I asked the nurses how much longer it would be before he went in for surgery. Although, I could have standed waiting longer for him to go into this major surgery, Kendryck was

very hungry and very fussy.

The nurse told me it would be a little longer because his surgeon was still in surgery with another baby. So, my dad and grandma said they would take my place for a little while so I could go downstairs and outside for a few minutes to get some fresh air. I really didn't want to leave him but I knew I needed a break and the nurse said it would still be a little while before they came to get him.

It wasn't as long as we expected though. My mom and I were downstairs for about 3 minutes when my dad started calling my cell phone. He said the nurse just came in and told them they would be taking Kendryck to the holding room shortly. I panicked. I thought I wouldn't get there in time and they would go ahead and take him back. I mean, I had already signed all the consent papers so there was nothing stopping them.

Mom and I raced back inside and had to wait in a VERY long line at the elevators. I contemplated taking the stairs but that was 15 flights of stairs and I would still be arriving around the same time. I think it was the 3rd elevator we were finally able to get on.

When we were back on the 15th floor, I raced to Kendryck's room. The closer I got, the more I could tell the unidentified male voices were coming from his room. I ran faster. As I entered the room, I didn't even say anything to anyone. I just went to my grandma and took Kendryck from her. I felt bad later, but I needed to hold him then.

It was time to go to the holding room. I could only choose one person to go with me and I couldn't decide to bring my mother or my father. So my father took a stand and said he was going. My heart was saddened as my mom kissed Kendryck and I cried because I wanted her to be with him, too, but deep inside, I knew Mom couldn't be as strong as Dad could in this situation. He knew I needed someone to hold me up when the time came.

Since Kendryck was awake and fussy, they allowed me to hold him instead of wheeling him upstairs in the bed. We were just moving up a couple of floors, but he wanted his mommy and his mommy wanted him so that was that.

Even more waiting came once we made it to the holding room. Kendryck was inconsolable. We turned cartoons on, I rocked him, we tried to play with him but he was so hungry and didn't understand why I wouldn't feed him.

Finally a different nurse brought me this

flavored water packet to dip his binky in. That seemed to do the trick. I gave Kendryck his binky and rocked him and before long, he was sleeping. Being able to hold him with him sleeping so good consoled me for a little while until I saw the man in the white coat appear. It was about 9:30 a.m. and it was time.

The man in the white coat was the anesthesiologist. He was going to administer some pre surgery meds to make Kendryck basically go into a deep sleep. He talked to us for a little while and was explaining what medicines he was administering and for what reasons.

There were two syringes. When, he started the first one in Kendryck's IV, Kendryck immediately woke up and looked around with terror in his eyes. Once again, he didn't know what was going on. But as he administered the rest of the medications, Kendryck went back to sleep. The anesthesiologist then said it was time to say our goodbyes. This threw me off.

Before I had been told that I would be able to hold Kendryck and carry him to the doors leading to the surgical room. But now that had changed. He took Kendryck out of my arms and said it was time. Just thinking about this makes me cry.

Remembering this moment is very painful for me. I wasn't sure if I would ever see my baby alive again. I still feel the pain I did that day when I had to say goodbye. I still remember and feel the emptiness and uncertainty I felt that morning.

I just kept kissing Kendryck on his little head and I whispered in his ear, "Be strong, my angel. Fight for Mommy. I'll be here waiting for you." And then when I said, "I love you," there it was. My second breakdown.

My legs felt weak and I thought I was going to collapse right there. The outbursts were uncontrollable. I couldn't hold the sobs and the more I tried, the louder they were. I watched until the anesthesiologist was all the way out of the room with my angel and the door closed. My dad just held me. I knew he was hurting, too, and I could see the pain and tears on his face but he just wanted to be there for me.

Chapter Six

After a few minutes, I told Dad I wanted to get out of there. We grabbed the bags we had and went to the room the young lady had shown us before where we were to wait while he was in surgery.

Someone would be giving us updates periodically about how his surgery was going and if there were any complications. Just hearing the word "complications" made me want to vomit (sorry for the bluntness).

The lady at the front desk informed me that it would be at least 30 minutes to an hour before we got the first update so Dad thought it wise that we go downstairs and meet up with my mom and other family who had came for support so we could get some fresh air.

As soon as I rounded the corner and saw my mom, two of my cousins, and a dear friend standing there, I started crying again. My cousin wrapped me in her arms and held me tight while I cried and before I knew it, I had several sets of arms around me. I am grateful to them for coming that day. I needed all the support I could get and they gave plenty of it.

While we were standing there, my maternal grandmother pulled in with her friend and her friend's daughter to lend more support. I can't express enough how grateful I was to everyone who was there. I don't think I could have done this on my own. Actually, I know I couldn't do this on my own. This was simply too hard. No one ever wants to see their baby get taken away by a doctor so they can operate on their heart... or on anything for that matter.

Soon after, I returned back upstairs and waited for an update. An hour later I still hadn't heard anything so I went to ask the lady at the front desk if she had. She replied that she hadn't but she would call up and find out what was going on.

She did this while I was standing there and then said, "Someone is coming down to speak to you," and then directed me to go to a holding room.

So, through any experience I had with any doctor, the only news they didn't give over the phone was bad news. Waiting patiently was not an option after this. I just knew they were going to come to give me bad news. I couldn't sit still. I bounced around impatiently, walked back and forth, and sighed quite a bit.

A lady in a t-shirt and scrubs came in. She had a cell phone attached to her and I think she had a clipboard. The nurse sat down across from us and started to speak. As soon as she did, the cell phone rang. It was information on my son's surgery.

She hung the phone up and told me they had Kendryck opened up and he was on the bypass machine, which meant his heart wasn't beating anymore. This device was keeping his blood and oxygen pumping and threw him like a replacement heart.

Just the thought of my baby lying on an operating table with his chest cut open and his heart not beating made me cringe. More fear grew inside me. The lady assured me that everything was going good. No complications. That part relieved me.

I returned to the waiting area but couldn't

keep my mind off of my sweet Kendryck. I couldn't

sit still either. My mom went downstairs and bought

me an iced coffee. I didn't want to go downstairs

incase she came back out with another update. At

one point I had to, though.

The day before the surgery, the social

worker returned like she promised and told me

about this assistance that Kendryck's insurance did.

I had never heard of it before. They would wire me

money for food for the extent of our stay at the

hospital.

So, I had to leave to go across the street and

pick it up. Since I was Kendryck's only guardian, I

was the only one who could sign for it. I wasn't

gone long though. After receiving the money, I

headed back to the hospital.

There was a coffee shop on the way. Since I

couldn't eat because of my nerves and I was absolutely exhausted, I stopped quickly to get a coffee to go and headed back.

It was about two hours before I got the next update. People always say no news is good news but I wasn't happy with that.

While waiting, I went into one of the restrooms and locked the door. Being in there, alone, made me silently reflect on what was going on and how my faith had dwindled quickly when I found out my son wasn't responding to medication.

I hit my knees there in the restroom, crying out to God for help... Begging Him to save my son, to save his heart. I begged for forgiveness and ask that God not hold it against my son for my dumb mistakes. I wondered if my faith hadn't dwindled if Kendryck had been healed before surgery. It was too late to take it back now. All I could do was move forward and hope and yes, pray, that Kendryck would survive.

I also prayed for God to guide the surgeon's hands and work through him to heal my baby. As I was praying, I had a sort of flashback, remembering what the surgeon had said before at the initial consultation. He informed me that before each surgery he prays to have God use his hands to help the child. He also said that he plays Christian music in the room while he's performing the surgery. Maybe that was God's way of reassuring me that He was already there.

After my third breakdown, I returned to the lady at the front desk inquiring about the status on Kendryck's surgery. I told her I hadn't heard anything in two hours and it was driving me crazy, to say the least.

Again, she called and had someone come give me an update. The update wasn't as long this time. She just reported that he was doing good still. There were still no complications. I wanted more information but she said they were still in the process of fixing his heart defects. I had to settle with that.

During the entire wait, I drank five very large coffees and walked probably five miles just in that little room. I tried reading but I couldn't consentrate. I tried to laugh but I felt guilty. I tried to rest but I couldn't. I was just so uneasy.

"It's My Heart" had brought me a "care package." There was a dry erase board, a spiral notebook, some pens, a shirt, a drawstring bag, a sports bottle, and I can't remember what else. I even tried fiddling around with a few of those things but I was too distracted. I just wanted to hold my baby.

Finally the time came for the next update. Two hours later, they called my name and told me to wait in a consultation room. I, of course, brought my parents with me, as I did every time. My dad and I paced back and forth across the room as my mom tried to talk to us to keep us calm. It seemed to be an eternity before the lady in the scrubs returned.

When she did, she wasn't smiling and I thought for sure I had lost him. She sat down in a chair and sighed. Then she said, "Everything is finished and there are still no complications. The surgeon is wiring his chest back together now and then sewing him up." Those are not the exact words she used, but it's the basics. She said when the surgeon finished wiring his breastbone together and

sewing his chest back up, he would come talk to
me.

I returned to the waiting area and relayed
what she had said. I was so pleased that he made it
through the surgery, but we weren't in the clear yet.
Kendryck still had to start breathing on his own
again and we had to see if what the surgeon had
done in his heart would stay.

At the first consultation, the surgeon assured
me that Kendryck's surgery was relatively common.
There wasn't as much risk as what we thought and
there was a 99 percent chance he would never have
to have another surgery. But there was still a chance
that whatever he had done wouldn't work.

Most of my family left after I gave them this
information. It was about 3:30 when we had gotten
that update so it was getting late and they had

families to return to and a long drive at that.

My cousins, my friend, my maternal grandmother and her two guests left. Only two people could be in the CVICU room at a time and they knew I would be the first one up there, naturally, since I am his mother. And it would still be a while before anyone could see him so they decided it was best to go ahead and go. All who were left now were Mom, Dad, my paternal grandmother, and myself.

It was about 30 minutes before the surgeon came in. He came in with a smile showing the brightest, whitest teeth I think I have ever seen. He said in fact, Kendryck's surgery went great but now we had to play the waiting game again. Kendryck was on life support and had to start breathing on his own and, as I was told before, they had to make sure it would hold.

The surgeon explained there were four holes as they had suspected but the largest one that had seemed to be the size of a dime was actually the size of a nickel. That's a pretty big hole for a baby's heart. He explained that a baby's heart is supposed to be the size of a strawberry but Kendryck's heart was about 3 times that size.

He then proceeded to tell us what all he had done during the surgery. The two smaller holes were left alone because, as the cardiologist said, they didn't matter on their own. The smaller of the larger holes required a couple of stitches and the largest hole required a patch. Then he explained about the valve.

The surgeon said he had to cut through an aortic valve to get to the valve that was partially blocked. He simply shaved off the excess tissue and stitched the aortic valve back up.

The surgeon thanked me for allowing him to perform the surgery on my baby. I thanked him for allowing God to work through him and saving my baby's life. I loved the fact that he gave God all the credit.

I asked him if I could see Kendryck and he told me it would be a few minutes because they were getting him transferred to and set up in the CVICU but someone would come get me when he was ready.

Finally, I could breathe. I had a sense of relief and peace rush through my veins because the surgery was over. Those 5 hours was like living an eternity in hell on earth.

But that had passed now and he made it

through surgery. I felt as is God was rejuvenating me and giving me the strength for the obstacles we still had to face.

Now I could willingly walk downstairs and get some fresh air without feeling so much fear. I took this time to call and text people to let them know Kendryck was out of surgery and everything went great. My baby had survived surgery and now I was ready to tackle the next trial because I knew God was by our side.

Chapter Seven

When I returned upstairs, it was time to see my strong, sleeping angel. The lady at the front desk directed me how to get there and my mother accompanied me. I was excited to finally get to see him but scared at what I was going to see, too.

When I entered the CVICU, I asked a nurse which room Kendryck was in and she pointed to where I needed to go. I raced to the door but stopped abruptly as I reached it. There were three babies in the room. Two of them were too small to be Kendryck but the third baby didn't look like my son at all.

I guess I wasn't really prepared for what I was going to see. There was a baby lying on the bed with no shirt on. His chest had a long strip of gauze over it, taped down securely. He had a tube coming out of his side and he was restrained to the bed.

There was an IV line in his wrist and one in his

neck and there was still an IV in his hand and foot.

He had a device wrapped around his head to

measure brain activity and he was on life support.

There were many lines and machines everywhere

but the one thing that stood out to me the most was

that this baby's chest did not cave in and his head

did not move when a breath of air was pushed into

his tiny body.

This could not be my son. I had known this

baby for 4 days shy of 7 months and his chest had

always caved in. But this was my baby. This was

my son attached to all these machines and gadgets

and not moving at all.

Standing in the door looking at him, I

thought I had lost him. I thought he had joined the

team of angels in the sky because there was no evidence of any life in him. As I got closer though, I could see his chest rise with each push of air.

The tears welled up in my eyes again as I watched him lying there, motionless. I touched his little arm and his skin was cold. This was new to me, too. In his almost seven months of life, Kendryck had never once been cold. His body worked too hard for each breath so he stayed warm, like he was constantly exercising.

The nurse was young, my age, maybe a little older. She explained to me everything that was going on.

There was one line for blood transfusions, that were currently being administered. His eyes were sunken in and dark because he needed more blood.

The other lines were for antibiotics that are necessary after surgery to fight infections.

Of course, the lines in his nose and strapped to his beautiful face was the ventilator. The ventilator was what was keeping him alive. Since he was on the lung-bypass machine during surgery, he basically had to relearn how to breathe on his own again.

The nurse went through everything with me. She showed me the numbers on the ventilator. There were numbers that looked like 20/20 which resembled how many breaths he was taking and how many breaths the machine was giving. So he was taking 20 breaths and the machine was administering all 20 of them.

I found myself staring at this machine relentlessly, just hoping for him to take one breath on his own.

Seconds went by, then minutes and hours and still no breaths on his own. It frightened me that he hadn't taken a breath on his own yet. I sat by his bed except for a couple of short breaks, one to get some fresh air and stretch, and one to eat because my parents seemed to think I needed to. Then, I was back by his side.

The social worker came in and informed me that I was given a room from the Ronald McDonald house but I needed to go sign in before they closed the front desk.

Dad and my grandma went upstairs to be with Kendryck so Mom and I could go take care of that. Someone showed us the room and, though I was really thankful, I had a sudden sense of sadness. I didn't want to be that far away from

Kendryck. It was all the way downstairs, across the driveway to the other building, and down deep in some winding hallways.

They had given us a key to be able to get in and out when we needed to but it was still too far away from me. On the walk back, I told my mom that she and my dad could have the room. After all, I felt I owed it to them because they were constantly right there by my side.

They did protest quite a bit, saying that I needed to rest and such, but nothing they said worked. I wasn't going to even take a chance at being that far away from him.

I told my parents I would sleep there in the lobby so I could get back to him quickly. There were tons of people in there but they were all sleeping, too, and the chairs were very comfortable.

I went back up to see Kendryck before trying to get some sleep. The CVICU room was too small and they wouldn't allow parents to sleep in there. As usual, I argued. I argued that I would just stay up all night then. I didn't want to leave him.

But the nurse on this shift was an older woman, a mother and grandmother, so she was patient with me. Plus, she had been doing this for years and she probably saw it with every set of parents that had a baby in this situation.

She said that Kendryck would be waking up sometime the next day and he needed to see his mommy's face. This did me in. It was settled. I would go down to the lobby and sleep for a few hours, if possible, and then I would return by his side.

I sat there for a little while. The nurse said I

could take my time saying goodnight, so I did.

Again, I kept watching the screen attached to the ventilator. No change. But then suddenly, the machine was showing 21/20, which meant he had taken a breath on his own. I like to think this was God's way, and Kendryck's, too, of showing me that he was okay for now and I could get some rest.

So, I kissed Kendryck goodnight with the same technique I had used every time he slept since the day he was born. It started with three kisses on the forehead (three kisses symbolize, "I love you"), then I would say, "Sweet dreams, Angel, Mommy loves you," and then one last kiss to seal the deal.

I'm not exactly sure why I did this, but I had done it since he was born and it stuck. And I definitely wasn't about to stop now.

Once I had kissed him goodnight, I started

downstairs and called my mother, who was already
at the Ronald McDonald house with my father. I
had to tell her the good news of Kendryck taking his
first breath on his own. It was now a little after
midnight.

After talking to Mom, I curled up in a chair
with a blanket and tried to get some sleep. And
sleep, I did. I experienced a bit of guilt when I woke
up and it was 6 a.m. I rushed back up stairs to see
him.

When I arrived upstairs, I saw the team of
doctors making their rounds. Luckily, they hadn't
been to Kendryck's room yet.

I rushed by his side and he was still sleeping
but something had changed. The ventilator screen
showed 26/20. He was now taking 6 breaths on his
own and he was starting to move. I could tell by the

look on his face, though, he was in pain.

It was only a few minutes before the team of doctors made it to Kendryck's bed. They explained to me that they wanted him to fully wake up so they could take him off of life support.

Once they had him fully awake, off of the venitlator and the lines out of his neck and wrist, I could finally hold my son. I was like a little kid at Christmas. I couldn't wait to hold him again.

It seemed to take forever for the day to progress and for me to be able to hold him but that time finally came. I had to leave his room so they could take the tube out of his nose and the IV lines out of his arteries so I took this time to take a shower and drink a coffee.

When I was allowed to go back in, he looked like a totally different baby. The big machine was out of his face, the lines were out (excluding the original ones in his hand and foot for the antibiotics) and the contraption around his head was gone.

There was one single oxygen line across his face, wrapped around his ears, and two adhesive patches to hold them down on each side of his face.

He was sleeping sound and was covered with a new blanket, red and blue with sports pictures and teddy bears all over. The flip side of the blanket had hearts all over it. I was told it was from an organization who donate them to the CVICU for the babies after surgery. Yet another reason to be grateful.

I didn't hold him at first because I had to wait for a nurse to take him out of the bed and hand him to me and because he was sleeping so good.

Waking him was not an option to me. He needed his rest.

It didn't take too long for him to wake up and I was right there when he did. I felt blessed that his eyes were open and he was looking for his mommy. I felt blessed that, so far, he had survived. And I had a sense of peace that things would go smoothly in the days to come and he would overcome the obstacles and trials set in his path.

I sat in the chair by his bed, scared and impatient at the same time, and the nurse moved all his wires around carefully. I was afraid I would hurt him or accidentally tug at a wire but she assured me I would do just fine.

At last, my baby boy was in my arms again and it felt great. I sat there examining him like I had done the first time I was able to really hold him after his birth.

The doctors had taken the gauze off of his incision and it was clearly visible. The surgeon had done the stitches on the inside somehow so you couldn't really tell they were even there. There were small strips of tape going across it all the way down and iodine covered the entire cut.

The chest tube was also still in place. It was a tube that went in right under his ribs and went up and around his heart. This is how the excess fluid was drained from inside.

Since I was afraid of hurting Kendryck when I held him, the nurse instructed me on how to hold him so that no pain would be caused.

There was a little baby next to Kendryck in the CVICU who was just a few months younger. His mommy was getting to hold him today, too. The only difference was this was the first time she held him since he was a few weeks old. He had been in the hospital for that long.

The other baby's mother and grandmother and I became friends and I would bring him balloons when I brought Kendryck's and we all would sit and talk for hours. Although we live so far away, we still talk from time to time and the grandma sends me pictures of her growing grandson who is now a happy, healthy toddler bouncing around everywhere.

This day in the CVICU was a bittersweet day for both of us moms. We both held our babies that day. I hold that family close to my heart and forever will.

Though I wished I could hold Kendryck forever, I couldn't. His little body just wasn't ready for it. So the nurse returned him to his bed.

Later in the night, he was allowed to eat for the first time since midnight before surgery. I knew he was happy about this. But they would only give him two ounces of formula to start out with since it had been so long since he ate anything.

Kendryck took that in in about a minute or two and he wanted more. Fortunately, the nurse said she could give him baby food because it was solid and he would probably be able to hold it down better. She left for a short time to get one of the feeder bottles. The nurse fed Kendryck because she knew the signs to look for incase he aspirated. He ended up eating the 2 ounces of formula and 2 jars of baby food.

Kendryck was content then. He went to sleep and it was time for me to go back down to the lobby to try and sleep. The nurse said they would probably move him to a regular room the next day and my momma duties were back on so I needed to get my rest tonight.

The lady at the front desk in the lobby gave me a card key like doctors and nurses use to get up and down the elevator after hours. This way, I could go see Kendryck anytime I wanted. I guess it gave me even more peace knowing I could get to him anytime I needed to with no problems or hassles because I slept til 7 a.m.

I woke up to the sun shining in the large windows in the lobby and was filled with panic. I left my things there and ran to the elevator and to his bed to see him. But, of course, everything was still okay.

When my parents got there, I went back

downstairs to collect my things and get ready to

move to a regular room. I was confident he would

be moving that day.

Chapter Eight

Sure enough Kendryck was doing well enough to be moved. The surgeon even made the comment, "Are you sure I just operated on him?"

He said Kendryck was at the stage most babies are a few days later. He was already lifting himself off the bed and moving around really good. So there was no doubt he was ready to be moved.

The surgeon explained to me the chest tube would have to stay in while he was being transferred because there was still a great amount of fluid being drained. He said when the chest tube could come out, Kendryck would probably be discharged the next day.

That day, while still in the CVICU, my parents took over for a little while and a friend brought me some food because I had been eating fast food the whole time we were there and she thought I needed some real food. I thought so, too. It was nice and I was thankful for her, too.

Then it was my shift again. But when I had made it back up there, they were getting him ready to be moved.

They moved him to a holding room until his room on the 15th floor was ready. Kendryck slept and I was nearly asleep when the surgeon came in.

I loved how the surgeon didn't just come in at certain times during the day. He came in several times a day to check on my son. And he came to check on me, too.

Finally, we were moved to the 15th floor which as any mother of a heart patient will tell you, is a huge success.

The only problems were the constant drainage in his chest tube which hendered having it removed, and the constipation from all the medication. One night he vomited all over his incision, and since I'm sure it hurt, he wasn't happy. But I held him and bounced and sang to him until he went back to sleep and all was good.

I was instructed on how to hold him. I had to re-learn holding an infant basically. You know, holding one hand under the bottom and one hand behind the head. But doing this with a 7 month old was quite difficult. I couldn't lift him under his arms either because it could rip his incision back open.

The days all ran together. Kendryck became more and more playful each day. One day, the nurse on that certain shift, told me about the room down the hallway with little wagons in them. She said I could take Kendryck for a ride around the "heart floor."

By this time, Kendryck wasn't hooked to any more machines. He was off of the oxygen and the IV poles were disconnected. He still had the IV's in his hand and foot for when they administered the medications, and he still had the chest tube.

He loved the ride. We visited his friend who was next to him in CVICU who had finally been moved to the 15th floor.

Each day he seemed to progress. One day a doctor came in and said it was time to take the chest tube out. My dad decided he would be the one to stay upstairs because he knew I couldn't stand to see him in pain anymore.

First, they came in to give a pain medication

but both of his IV's had slipped out his hand and foot so the liquid spilled out. I think they ended up giving him a shot.

I hadn't been gone for five minutes when Dad called me. I know I hadn't even made it downstairs. Dad reported that the tube was out and they had put a suture in. He said as soon as they had the suture in, Kendryck put his toe in his mouth and bit it for the first time. He also said that he was doing great and only whined when he bit his toe.

The next day, another chest x-ray and echocardiogram were done. With the echocardiogram, they showed me where the patch was in his heart but I was most pleased because there was no blood backflowing.

However, there was more fluid around his heart so he had to remain on two medications, excluding the pain meds.

That day, Kendryck was discharged from the hospital and his insurance company paid for us to stay in a hotel room for three days until his appointment for his check-up.

The days in the hotel room went slowly but it was nice quality time. We played games and watched tv, but most of all, we enjoyed that Kendryck was with us happy and laughing.

On the third day, we returned to the hospital for his check-up. I was told Kendryck weighed 16.9 pounds, when the morning of surgery just 9 days earlier, he weighed 15.2 pounds. He was finally gaining. He had also went from 0 to 3 months clothes to 6 to 9 months clothes in that week and went from a size 2 diaper to a size 3. He was in fact, growing.

Kendryck was doing great. There wasn't much fluid left so there was no need for anymore medications. His incision was already healing and the tape was falling off one by one, and he had the suture removed where his chest tube was.

We were sent home the day before Halloween and told to follow up with the cardiologist in a few weeks.

On this visit with the cardiologist, my mom had to work so my dad accompanied us. I was confident Kendryck was doing great. He was starting to sit up on his own and trying to start flipping on his belly again.

The doctor said not to put him on his belly for 6 weeks but if he rolled over, it was okay for him to stay that way for a few minutes. It was about 8 weeks total before he could be on his belly freely, so he was a little behind with his tummy time and crawling.

Although I was confident Kendryck was doing great, there was still a fear deep inside. From talking to other mom's who have been through this journey, or something similar, I learned that that fear is always there.

The same tests were ran only this time, my son didn't turn to me for comfort, he wanted his PawPaw. He loves his grandparents like another set of parents.

When the tests were all done, the cardiologist met us in an exam room and explained that the fluid was building back up. There was a tremendous amount of fluid around Kendryck's heart again and if they couldn't get it cleared up with medication, they would have to make a small incision (similar to the incision for the chest tube) under his ribs and drain the fluid.

I'm not going to lie. I was mortified. Could he be starting all over? Could our journey just start all over that easily after all the trials and tests we had already overcome?

I was mainly scared for Kendryck. He had been through so much and had went from being so tiny and fragile to being a growing, healthy boy. He had become so strong and was progressing very quickly. I didn't want all of this to end for him.

The cardiologist prescribed steroids to decrease the fluid around his heart. This time, however, I wasn't going to abandon my faith as I did before. The first thing I did was pray. I mean strong, meaningful prayer.

The following Sunday, Mom, Kendryck, and

I went to church together and I brought Kendryck to the front for prayer. I explained the situation and everyone in the church surrounded him.

We all prayed for a long time, hoping that our prayers would be heard and Kendryck wouldn't have to go through any other surgeries or anything. We prayed for God to just heal him. And that, He did.

The follow-up visit with the cardiologist was a rewarding one. Once again, the same tests were ran and the cardiologist came back in with a smile. He proudly announced there was only a tiny bit of fluid left and in a few days it would all be gone. No more medications and no cardiology visits for six months! And that was that!

Chapter Nine

After the surgery, I would stare at him and wonder if this was some fluke. If this was supposed to happen. Was it a mistake or some kind of punishment to me? I had a difficult time dealing with all the emotions.

Late at night, I would lay next to him, wide awake, and just cry. I would whisper to him and say, "Thank you for fighting, Baby. Thank you for staying here with Mommy. I don't know what I'd do without you, or how I'd make it."

Every moment with him is bittersweet. I have recorded his laughter and him saying, "Mama" and set them as ringtones on my phone. I wake everyday to see his face. I take each breath because he has breath in his tiny body. I think more, I smile more, I live more.

Kendryck is a miracle and I am so blessed to have him as my son. He has made me a better person in the short time I have had him in my life.

I know each day that I am lucky, and blessed, that Kendryck is still here with me. I've read the statistics. I've seen the youtube videos of babies who didn't survive. I know that if it weren't for God and the amazing medical team who took care of my baby, he could have easily joined that team of Angel Babies in Heaven.

I can't tell you how saddened I am to see a picture of a baby who didn't survive Congenital Heart Disease, or any disease for that matter. When I watch the videos, I cry relentlessly because I know what they were feeling. I've sat by my baby's hospital bed, with tubes and wires hooked all over him, and had the thoughts that my baby may not make it.

I also can't tell you how many nights I was so scared to go to sleep because I was worried Kendryck wouldn't open his eyes the next morning.

So, when I watch these videos, I know their pain and I just want to reach out to them. I want to hold each and every one of them, parents and babies, and let them know someone is there for them. Someone cares. I care.

Maybe, "Everything happens for a reason," is true. Maybe God did place these obstacles in our lives so that we could be a living, walking testimony to other parents and children going through the same hardships of this deadly disease. Maybe God knew that Kendryck and I would be good at helping people going through the same struggles we endured.

I don't know for sure why God chose to add Kendryck to the never ending list of babies who are diagnosed with CHD, but I know that wallowing in sadness because he went through that is not the answer. Yes, Kendryck had a lot of pain and tons of medical problems, and I hate that he had to go through that. Nevertheless, he overcame. We both did.

He was here to celebrate his 1st Halloween (the day after we came home), his 1st Thanksgiving (8 months), his 1st Christmas (9 months), and his 1st Birthday, another whole year full of holidays, and his 2nd Birthday! Today, Kendryck is 2 years and 9 months old.

We have also incorporated a kind of second

birthday. October 21st. The day Kendryck had open heart surgery and survived.

Each year we have a little celebration to thank God for healing his little heart. As he gets older, each celebration will grow. Not just because he's getting older, but because it's another year added to his "Survivor Time."

Today, Kendryck is doing great. He still has two small holes in his heart but they are expected to grow up by the time he's 5.

Kendryck had his last cardiology appointment on March 29th, 2010. His cardiologist informed me that there's no need for him to come back for 2 years! That is a major accomplishment.

Today, Kendryck is 38 pounds and about 40 inches tall! He has blonde, crazy curls and he still has those big beautiful blue eyes. He runs and plays just like any other kid and he is very smart. He loves to learn.

He, of course, still has the scar from his surgery and a scar from the chest tube, but they're barely noticeable. But if you meet Kendryck, and you've never seen his scar, he'll voluntarily show you. It's his "Battle Scar." He loves to show it off.

Kendryck is a loving baby. He loves to give people hugs and kisses. I don't think Kendryck has ever met a stranger. He will walk through stores shaking all the men's hands and blowing kisses to all the ladies. He is great to other kids, too. Kendryck loves when he is around another kid, whether they're his age or not. There's no other way to explain it, except he's just a loving baby.

October 21st, 2010 was 2 years since

Kendryck's surgery, and since he became a survivor in my book. It's hard to explain the satisfaction of knowing your baby is going to be okay.

Meeting those "mile markers" gives the greatest feelings imaginable. Still, every time he has to go to his pediatrician, I hold my breath when he listens to his heart and lungs. I am constantly afraid we're going to go one day and the doctor is going to tell me Kendryck's heart problems are back. But a mother always worries, right?

Okay, it is time for me to end this but before I go, I would like to ask you to please read up on Congenital Heart Disease and spread awareness. You could end up telling someone about CHD who just found out their child has it and doesn't know anything about it.

Also, I ask to always remember how special your child is. Love them with all of your being and more. Kids are a gift from God and some become angels too soon. You never know what's going to happen, or when, so make sure your child, or children, know you love them.

Make sure you, and your child, or children, live each day to the fullest together and make sure to give God thanks for giving your baby, or babies, to you.

Thank you for sharing our journey with us. We hope that, in some way, we helped you in some aspect of your life. Please share this book with anyone you think can benefit from it. And please always live, laugh, pray, and love. God bless you all and may he keep you wrapped with in His

everlasting love. I wish you all the best!

Krystal

Mom of a SURVIVOR!

In honor of Kendryck!

In loving memory of
"Nannie"
Nadean Taylor Phillips
3/1/1929 – 09/19/10
Please continue to hold our
hands and guide us
through our good and bad
times as you did in life. I
love you. Always have.
ALWAYS will!

www.ingramcontent.com/pod-product-compliance
Lightning Source LLC
Chambersburg PA
CBHW072143280526
45788CB00002B/762